The Visual Guide to

Asperger's Syndrome in 8-11 Year Olds

by Alis Rowe

Also by Alis Rowe

One Lonely Mind
978-0-9562693-0-0

The Girl with the Curly Hair - Asperger's and Me
978-0-9562693-2-4

The 1st Comic Book
978-0-9562693-1-7

The 2nd Comic Book
978-0-95626934-8

The 3rd Comic Book
978-0-9562693-3-1

The 4th Comic Book
978-15086839-7-1

Websites:
www.alisrowe.co.uk
www.thegirlwiththecurlyhair.co.uk
www.womensweightlifting.co.uk

Social Media:
www.facebook.com/thegirlwiththecurlyhair
www.twitter.com/curlyhairedalis

The Visual Guide to

Asperger's Syndrome in 8-11 Year Olds

by Alis Rowe

Lonely Mind Books
London

Copyrighted Material

Published by
Lonely Mind Books
London

First edition 2014
Second edition 2015

Printed and bound in the USA

For parents and teachers of children with Asperger's Syndrome

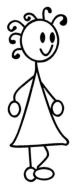

hello

This guide is all about 8 to 11 year old girls with Asperger's Syndrome and other Autism Spectrum Disorders (ASD).

Some of the information may also be applicable to boys.

It contains challenges that are common to children with ASD, and suggested ways to deal with these challenges at home and at school.

With thanks to Beccie Orchard for her real life insight as a parent.

I hope you enjoy this book.

Alis aka The Girl with the Curly Hair

Contents

AT THIS AGE, DIFFERENCES ARE BECOMING APPARENT MOSTLY BECAUSE OTHER CHILDREN THE SAME AGE AS THE GIRL WITH THE CURLY HAIR ARE MAKING FRIENDS EASILY (USUALLY FRIENDS OF THE SAME SEX)

THE GIRL WITH THE CURLY HAIR MAY WANT TO MAKE FRIENDS BUT SHE DOESN'T KNOW HOW TO. IT DOESN'T COME NATURALLY TO HER AND SHE FEELS LIKE THERE'S A BIG GAP BETWEEN HER AND HER PEERS...

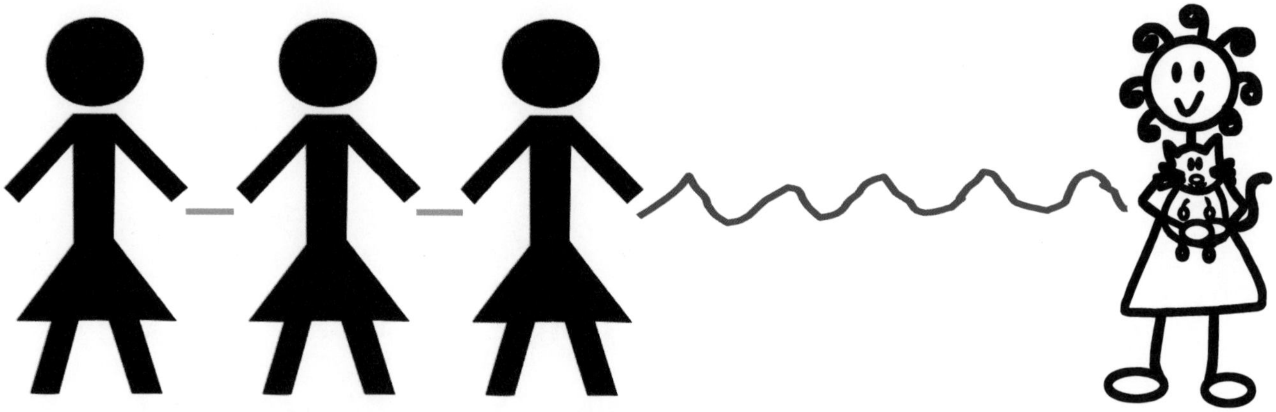

IN PARTICULAR, COMMUNICATING AND COOPERATING WITH OTHERS IS DIFFICULT

WHY IS COMMUNICATING AND COOPERATING WITH OTHERS HARD WORK FOR THE GIRL WITH THE CURLY HAIR?

SOMETIMES I WANT TO PLAY WITH MY CLASSMATES BUT I DON'T KNOW HOW TO

IF I'M NOT INTERESTED IN SOMETHING, FOR EXAMPLE WHAT MY FRIEND IS SAYING, I WILL JUST 'SWITCH OFF' COMPLETELY

I DON'T LIKE LOSING GAMES AND I END UP EITHER HAVING A TANTRUM OR A MELTDOWN. SOMETIMES I WON'T TALK OR EVEN ACKNOWLEDGE ANYONE FOR A LONG TIME AFTER LOSING

I ONLY REALLY LIKE OTHER CHILDREN IF THEY LIKE THE SAME THINGS AS ME

I CAN TALK FOR A LONG TIME ABOUT MY FAVOURITE THINGS, EVEN IF OTHERS AREN'T LISTENING

I CAN BE A CHARACTER AND PLAY WITH OTHERS BUT ONLY IF THEY TELL ME WHAT TO DO. I CAN'T WORK OUT WHAT TO DO IF I'M NOT TOLD EXACTLY

I CAN'T DO RECIPROCAL CONVERSATION AND I SEEM TO TALK "AT" PEOPLE RATHER THAN "WITH" THEM

I CAN'T ACCEPT THAT THE IDEA OF A BALL GAME IS FOR EVERYONE TO HAVE A GO WITH THE BALL AT SOME TIME

SOMETIMES I WON'T PLAY WITH ANYONE BECAUSE THE OTHERS DON'T DO AS I SAY

15

WHEREAS OTHER CHILDREN FAVOUR GROUP PLAY, CLUBS AND TEAM SPORTS...

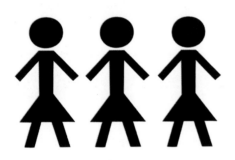

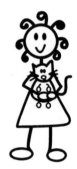

...SHE TENDS TO BE CONTENT ON HER OWN

WHAT ARE SOME OF HER FAVOURITE THINGS TO DO ON HER OWN?

I LIKE READING BOOKS

I LOVE DRAWING PICTURES

I LIKE PLAYING ON MY COMPUTER

I LIKE MAKING MY OWN BOARD GAMES WITH PAPER AND PENS

I LIKE BEING OUTSIDE, CLIMBING TREES AND RUNNING AROUND

I LIKE COLLECTING THINGS THAT ARE GREEN

I LIKE SCIENCE, NUMBERS AND FACTS

I LOVE ANIMALS, ESPECIALLY MY CATS

She's hardly ever bored...

She reads

- Can't walk past words without reading them
- Even junk mail and leaflets that come through the door

She creates

- Invents board games
- Draws complex machines and structures
- Creates new levels for her favourite video games

She imagines

- Makes up stories and films inside her head

19

Motor skills

Her motor skills are less developed than her peers, which means she can't – or won't – do certain things

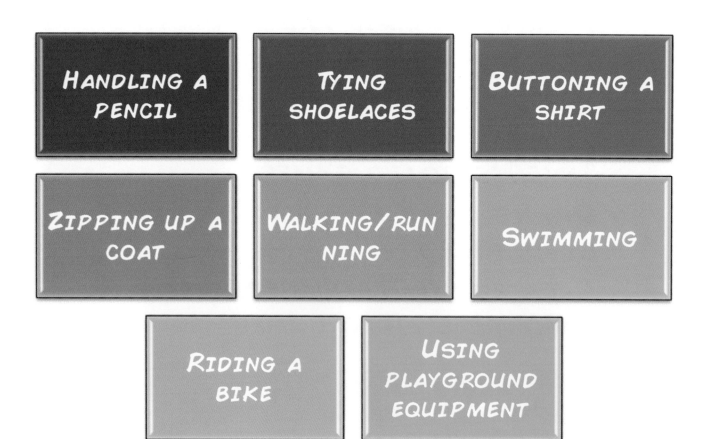

Handling a pencil	Tying shoelaces	Buttoning a shirt
Zipping up a coat	Walking/running	Swimming
Riding a bike	Using playground equipment	

She may be teased, bullied, or feel left out

Activities for developing motor skills

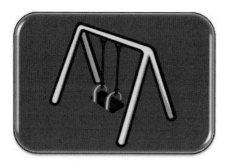

PLAYGROUND EQUIPMENT: SUPERVISED USE

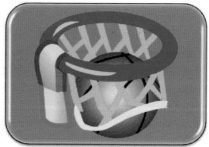

BASKETBALL: THROWING A BALL INTO A LOWERED HOOP

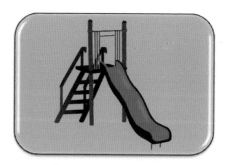

SLIDE LADDERS: CLIMBING WITH A GOAL

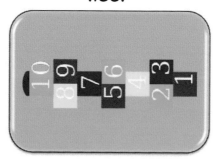

HOPSCOTCH: JUMPING OR SKIPPING INTO LARGE SQUARES

TREAT THESE IDEAS AS "PLAY" RATHER THAN "WORK". IF DONE WITH OTHERS, THEY MAY IMPROVE SOCIAL SKILLS AS WELL

LIFE AT HOME CAN BE HARD

EVEN IF PARENTS MAKE AN EFFORT TO UNDERSTAND ASD, LIFE AT HOME CAN STILL BE VERY DIFFICULT FOR CHILDREN WITH ASD

Why might life at home be hard for The Girl with the Curly Hair?

I'M NOT ALLOWED TO PLAY ON THE COMPUTER AS MUCH AS I WOULD LIKE TO

I CAN GET VERY CROSS WITH MY SISTER WHEN SHE DOESN'T DO WHAT I SAY. THIS CAN LEAD TO ME BEING AGGRESSIVE WITH HER

I CANNOT WAIT FOR ANYTHING, FOR EXAMPLE WHEN MUM IS DOING SOMETHING ELSE AND I WANT HER TO BE WITH ME. I GET VERY FRUSTRATED

MUM AND DAD SOMETIMES TELL ME THAT I AM BEING TOO LOUD, EVEN WHEN I AM ON MY OWN IN MY BEDROOM. THIS IS CONFUSING BECAUSE I DON'T THINK I'M BEING LOUD

I AM VERY FUSSY WITH FOOD. SOMETIMES, I REFUSE TO EAT MY DINNER IF I DON'T LIKE SOMETHING

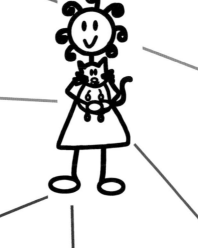

I DON'T LIKE HAVING BATHS OR BRUSHING MY TEETH. I OFTEN FEEL LIKE I AM BEING FORCED TO DO THESE WHEN I REALLY DON'T WANT TO

I DON'T LIKE WEARING CLOTHES, OTHER THAN MY PYJAMAS AND I GET STRESSED WHEN I'M ASKED TO "GET DRESSED"

I DON'T LIKE GOING TO BED. I JUST WANT TO STAY UP AND DO MY SPECIAL INTEREST

NOW LET'S GO THROUGH EACH OF THESE AND SEE HOW THE GIRL WITH THE CURLY HAIR THINKS EACH PROBLEM MAY BE SOLVED

PROBLEM: SHE WANTS EVERYTHING
HER WAY

SUGGESTION: REINFORCE THE CONCEPT OF TURN TAKING USING VISUALS AND SIGNS, E.G. WHEN IT'S HER TURN, THE HANGING SIGN IS BLUE (BE CREATIVE!)

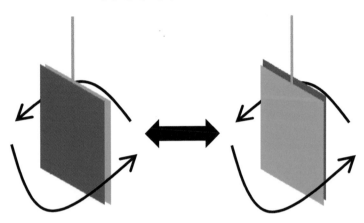

SUGGESTION: HAVE FILM OR GAME DAYS WHERE DIFFERENT FAMILY MEMBERS GET TO TAKE TURNS IN CHOOSING WHAT TO WATCH OR PLAY, ETC.

	MON	TUES	WED	THURS	FRI	SAT	SUN
FILM	TGWTCH	DAD	MUM	TGWTCH	DAD	MUM	TGWTCH
GAME	MUM	TGWTCH	DAD	MUM	TGWTCH	DAD	TGWTCH

SUGGESTION: TRY TO AVOID USING THE WORD "NO" DIRECTLY. INSTEAD, EMPHASISE THAT "YES WE CAN DO THAT *BUT* WE ARE GOING TO DO THIS *FIRST...*" OR "YES, NOT NOW, BUT LATER"

Problem: She makes very loud noises

THIS MAY BE A 'STIM', WHICH IS AN UNCONTROLLABLE OR UNCONSCIOUS WAY OF REGULATING ANXIETY. SOME CHILDREN HAVE AUDITORY PROCESSING PROBLEMS WHICH MEANS THEY ARE UNAWARE OF THEIR OWN VOLUME LEVEL

SUGGESTION: GENERALLY, STIMS THAT ARE NOT HARMFUL SHOULD BE ENCOURAGED AS THEY ARE ACTUALLY BENEFICIAL TO THE CHILD. HOWEVER, IF THE SOUND IS TOO LOUD, DISCUSS WITH HER APPROPRIATE SOUND LEVELS FOR DIFFERENT SETTINGS, E.G. AT HOME VS IN CHURCH. AGREE ON A SIGN, SUCH AS A NON-VERBAL SIGNAL OR AN ACTUAL SIGN, THAT CAN BE USED TO INFORM HER SHE IS BEING TOO LOUD

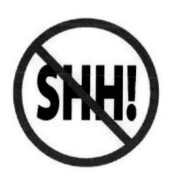 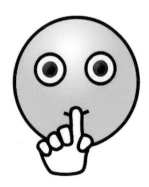

PROBLEM: SHE DOES NOT LIKE HAVING A BATH OR BRUSHING HER TEETH

SUGGESTION: EXPLAIN THE REASON WHY PERSONAL HYGIENE IS IMPORTANT

SUGGESTION: ALWAYS USE TOOTHPASTE OR BATH WASH THAT THE CHILD LIKES (EVEN IF YOU HAVE TO TRIAL A FEW INITIALLY)

SUGGESTION: ADAPT THE ENVIRONMENT, E.G. BUBBLE BATH, A TOY RELATING TO HER SPECIAL INTEREST, OR CANDLES (TAKE CARE!), COULD MAKE BATH TIME MORE ENJOYABLE FOR HER

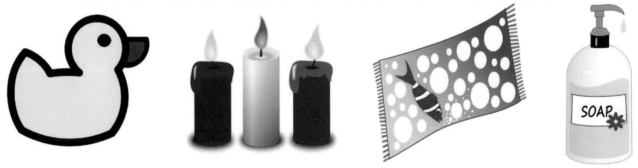

SUGGESTION: AN ELECTRIC OR BATTERY TOOTHBRUSH AS OPPOSED TO A MANUAL ONE COULD BE EASIER FOR THE CHILD TO HANDLE IF SHE HAS POOR MOTOR SKILLS. THE SENSORY EXPERIENCE IS LIKELY TO BE MORE CONSISTENT AND PREDICTABLE LEADING TO A SENSE OF COMFORT

PROBLEM: SHE DOES NOT LIKE GOING TO BED

SOME CHILDREN WITH ASD FIND SLEEPING A DISRUPTION OR AN ANNOYANCE THAT GETS IN THE WAY OF THEIR SPECIAL INTEREST

SUGGESTION: AGREE THAT, ONCE IN BED, SHE HAS X TIME TO DO HER SPECIAL INTEREST, E.G. PLAY ON THE COMPUTER, READ, LISTEN TO A STORY, ETC. *BEFORE* SLEEPING – BUT, THIS TIME IS ONLY GIVEN ONCE SHE IS ACTUALLY *IN* BED

SUGGESTION: GIVE THE CHILD THE FREEDOM TO DECORATE OR ARRANGE HER BEDROOM HOW SHE WANTS TO, WHICH WILL MAKE IT MORE LIKELY SHE'LL WANT TO GO TO BED

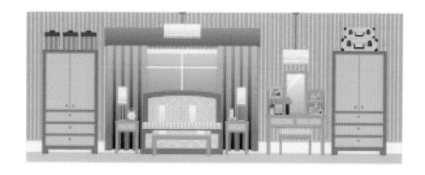

PROBLEM: SHE REFUSES TO GET DRESSED

CHILDREN WITH ASD MAY BE HIGHLY SENSITIVE TO THE FEEL OF CERTAIN FABRICS. NEVER FORCE THEM TO WEAR SOMETHING THEY FEEL UNCOMFORTABLE IN AS THIS CAN CAUSE DISTRESS

SUGGESTION: AGREE ON OUTFITS FOR OUT OF THE HOUSE THAT ARE BOTH PRESENTABLE AND COMFORTABLE, SUCH AS PLAIN JOGGING BOTTOMS

SUGGESTION: IN DRESS-SPECIFIC SITUATIONS, ADJUST THE OUTFIT IF POSSIBLE, E.G. A COTTON VEST CAN BE WORN DISCREETLY UNDERNEATH HER SCHOOL SHIRT

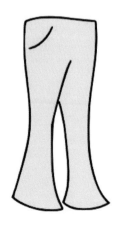

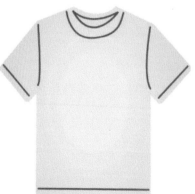

PROBLEM: SHE REFUSES TO EAT CERTAIN FOODS

TRY TO FIND OUT WHY. MANY CHILDREN WITH ASD ARE SENSITIVE TO APPEARANCE, TEXTURE OR SMELL OF FOOD. SOME DON'T LIKE DIFFERENT FOOD ITEMS TOUCHING EACH OTHER

SUGGESTION: ADAPT MEALS WHERE POSSIBLE SO THE CHILD CAN STILL JOIN IN WITH THE FAMILY MEAL, EVEN IF IT'S SERVED SLIGHTLY DIFFERENTLY

FOR EXAMPLE, "BEANS AND TOAST" – THE SAME MEAL CAN CERTAINLY BE SERVED IN MORE THAN ONE WAY...

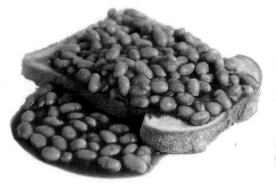
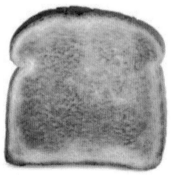
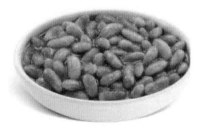

PROBLEM: SHE CANNOT WAIT/SHE HAS VERY LITTLE PATIENCE

SUGGESTION: MAKE SURE THINGS ARE EASILY AND READILY AVAILABLE SO THAT THE CHILD IS AS INDEPENDENT AS POSSIBLE, E.G. MAKE SURE THE LAPTOP IS ALWAYS CHARGED, READY MADE SNACKS ARE IN THE FRIDGE, ETC.

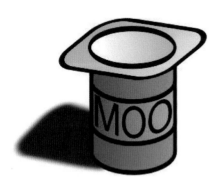 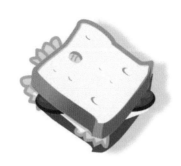 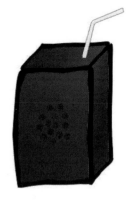

SUGGESTION:
IF THE CHILD IS WAITING ON ANOTHER PERSON, ENCOURAGE HER TO START THE TASK ON HER OWN UNTIL THE OTHER PERSON CAN JOIN IN, E.G. IF WAITING FOR MUM TO READ A BEDTIME STORY, MUM TELLS CHILD TO GO AND CHOOSE A BOOK UNTIL MUM IS READY

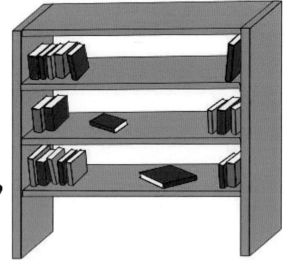

PROBLEM: SHE DOESN'T LIKE BEING TOLD TO GET OFF THE COMPUTER

SUGGESTION: COMPROMISE WITH THE CHILD ON WHAT IS BOTH 1) REALISTIC AND 2) SUFFICIENT TIME ON THE COMPUTER FOR HER TO DO WHAT SHE NEEDS TO DO

SUGGESTION: GIVE EXTRA COMPUTER TIME AS A REWARD FOR GOOD BEHAVIOUR

SUGGESTION: IF SHE HAS X TIME, USE A TIMER SO THAT SHE CAN SEE HOW MUCH TIME IS REMAINING AND CAN BE WARNED AS IT COMES TO AN END — IT WILL BE LESS DISRUPTIVE AND COME AS LESS OF A SURPRISE

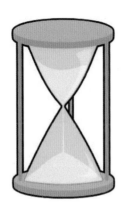 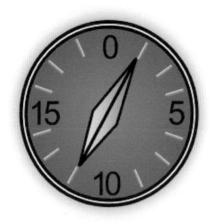 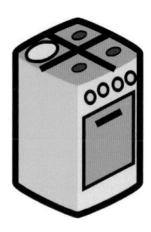

SCHOOL CAN BE INCREDIBLY HARD

NOW LET'S GO THROUGH SOME COMMON ASD CHALLENGES AND POSSIBLE SUGGESTIONS

(THE GIRL WITH THE CURLY HAIR SUGGESTS YOU SHOW THIS PART TO THE TEACHERS!)

PROBLEM: SHE CANNOT CONCENTRATE
ON SUBJECTS SHE FINDS DIFFICULT
OR ONES THAT DO NOT INTEREST
HER

SUGGESTION: SCHEDULE WORK SO THE STUDENT FEELS REWARDED BY A MORE ENJOYABLE TASK AFTER THE LESS ENJOYABLE TASK IS DONE, E.G.

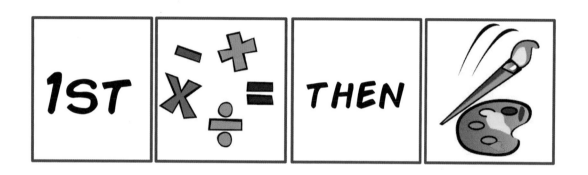

SUGGESTION: INCORPORATE THE STUDENT'S SPECIAL INTEREST (E.G. TRAINS) INTO THE TASK (E.G. MATHS), E.G. "THERE ARE FOUR TRAINS AT THE STATION. TWO DEPART. HOW MANY ARE IN THE STATION NOW?" USE DRAWINGS TOO

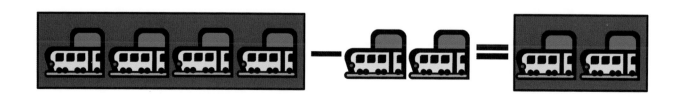

PROBLEM: SHE CANNOT STAY CALM WHEN SHE MAKES A MISTAKE – SHE IS VERY QUICKLY FRUSTRATED WHICH CAN QUICKLY TURN TO ANGER

SUGGESTION: BY COOPERATING WITH THE PARENTS, THE TEACHER CAN LEARN TO LOOK OUT FOR THE PHYSICAL SIGNS THAT INDICATE FRUSTRATION, E.G. HAND FLAPPING, ROCKING OR PACING

SUGGESTION: THE TEACHER AND THE STUDENT CAN AGREE ON A NUMBER OR COLOUR SYSTEM THAT ENABLES THE STUDENT TO COMMUNICATE HER LEVEL OF ANGER (MORE INFO ON PAGE 73...)

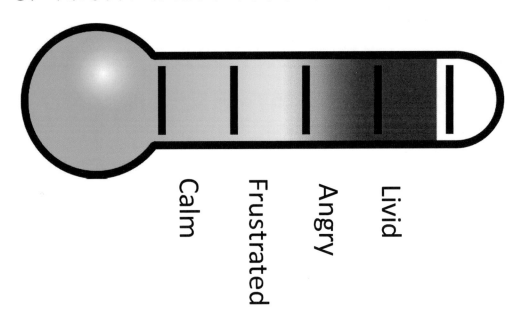

Calm — Frustrated — Angry — Livid

BEFORE "BOILING POINT" IS REACHED, THE TEACHER SIGNALS THAT IT'S BREAK TIME, E.G. FIVE MINUTES IN A QUIET ROOM, OR A GO ON THE SWINGS

PROBLEM: SHE CANNOT SUSTAIN FRIENDSHIPS OUTSIDE OF LESSONS, FOR EXAMPLE AT BREAK AND LUNCH TIMES

SUGGESTION: THE SCHOOL CAN CREATE A DEDICATED 'QUIET ROOM'

SUGGESTION: THE SCHOOL COULD SET UP LUNCH TIME INTEREST CLUBS, E.G. LEGO®, MINECRAFT®, READING

PROBLEM: SHE DOES NOT LIKE THE FOOD SERVED AT LUNCH TIME (AND THE OPTION OF A PACKED LUNCH IS NOT AVAILABLE)

SUGGESTION: A DETAILED WEEKLY MENU SHOULD BE ON DISPLAY IN ADVANCE OF THE WEEK, E.G.

MONDAY	TUESDAY	WEDNESDAY	THURSDAY	FRIDAY
CHICKEN BREAST, BROWN RICE AND PEAS				

SUGGESTION: FOR STUDENTS WHO HAVE TEXTURE SENSITIVITIES IN PARTICULAR, ALTERNATIVES SHOULD BE AVAILABLE AND THERE SHOULD ALWAYS BE A DEFAULT SELECTION OF 'PLAIN' OR UNTOUCHED FOODS, E.G.

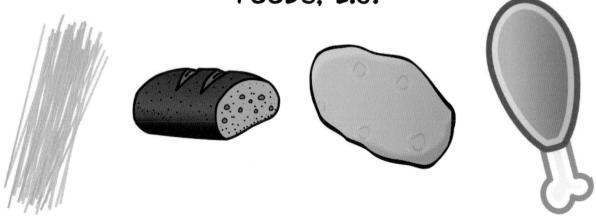

PROBLEM: SHE DOES NOT LIKE OTHER PEOPLE SITTING TOO CLOSE TO HER, PARTICULARLY DURING 'CIRCLE TIME' (SITTING ON THE FLOOR)

SUGGESTION: THERE COULD BE A CREATIVE GAME WHERE STUDENTS HAVE TO MAKE THEIR OWN 'PERSONAL SPACE' CIRCLES OUT OF PAPER OR PENS. ONLY THE EDGES OF THE CIRCLES ARE ALLOWED TO TOUCH:

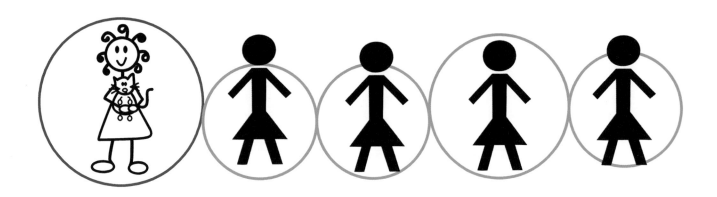

SUGGESTION: RATHER THAN SINGLE THE STUDENT OUT BY SEPARATING HER FROM EVERYONE ELSE, ALLOW ALL STUDENTS TO HAVE A SAY IN WHERE THEY SIT

PROBLEM: SHE CANNOT MANAGE HER ANXIETY ABOUT WHAT IS GOING TO HAPPEN NEXT IN THE LESSON

SUGGESTION: HAVE A SCHEDULE FOR EVERYONE TO SEE. THAT WAY, THE STUDENT WITH ASD CAN SEE A VISUAL OF HOW LONG THEY'VE GOT UNTIL A CHANGE IS GOING TO HAPPEN

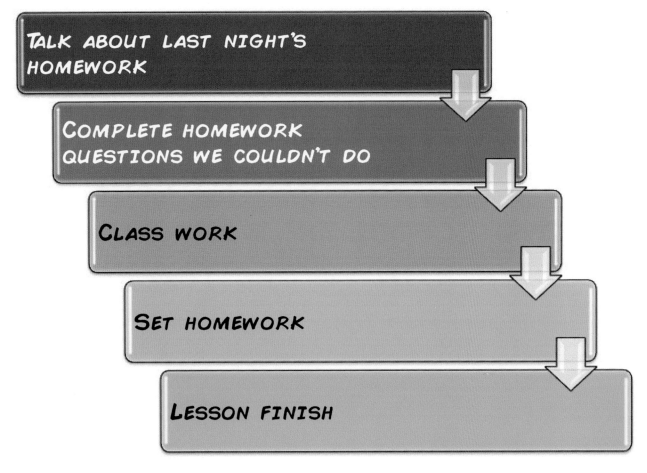

TALK ABOUT LAST NIGHT'S HOMEWORK

COMPLETE HOMEWORK QUESTIONS WE COULDN'T DO

CLASS WORK

SET HOMEWORK

LESSON FINISH

THEN THEY CAN TRY TO SELF-REGULATE WITHOUT ANXIETY ABOUT HOW LONG THEY HAVE TO DO EACH TASK FOR!

PROBLEM: SHE HAS TROUBLE REMEMBERING WHAT TO TAKE HOME FROM SCHOOL OR WHAT TO HAND BACK IN TO THE TEACHER

SUGGESTION: *THE TEACHER* COULD MAKE A LIST AT THE FRONT OF THE CLASS FOR THE WHOLE CLASS TO SEE. DRAWINGS ARE HELPFUL, E.G. A DRAWING OF A LETTER IN AN ENVELOPE THAT HAS TO BE TAKEN HOME

Take letter home

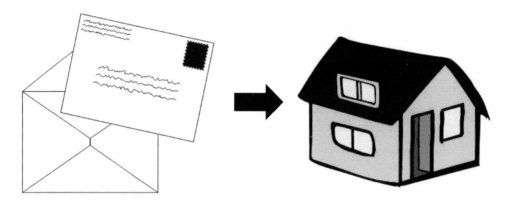

Return letter to school

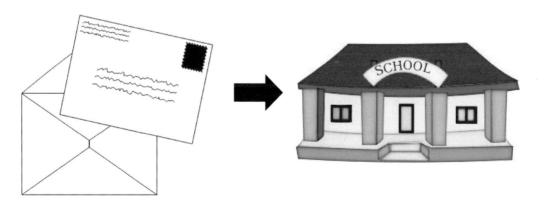

PROBLEM: SHE WILL NOT STOP FIDGETING IN CLASS

SINCE THIS IS TYPICALLY DUE TO A LACK OF CONCENTRATION, IT MAY HELP TO ALLOW THE STUDENT TO DO SOMETHING ELSE (USUALLY TACTILE) WHILST IN THE CLASS

HERE ARE SOME EXAMPLES OF THINGS:

A wobble cushion

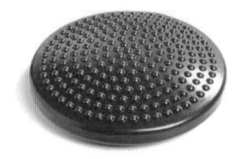

Chair bands

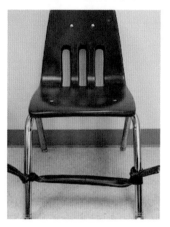

A weighted lap blanket

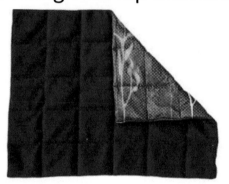

SCHOOLS SHOULD BE ABLE TO PROVIDE THESE UNDER THEIR SPECIAL EDUCATIONAL NEEDS (SEN) FUNDING

PROBLEM: SHE HAS VERY POOR HANDWRITING RELATIVE TO HER PEERS

THIS IS USUALLY CAUSED BY IMPAIRED FINE MOTOR SKILLS AND MAY MEAN THE STUDENT PRESENTS AS BEING "BELOW AVERAGE" IN THIS SKILL

SUGGESTION: PENCIL GRIPS SHOULD BE MADE AVAILABLE

SUGGESTION: MODERN TECHNOLOGY SHOULD BE EMBRACED. THE OCCASIONAL USE OF TABLET COMPUTERS, FOR CERTAIN TASKS, CAN REDUCE FRUSTRATION WITHOUT HER FEELING LEFT OUT

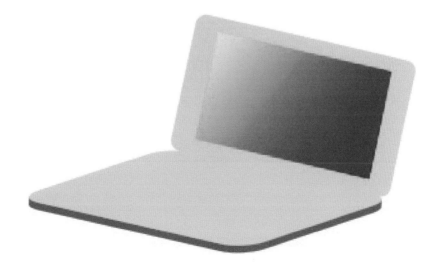

PROBLEM: : SHE ABSOLUTELY HATES P.E.

THIS IS LIKELY DUE TO TWO REASONS 1) PROBLEMS WITH GROSS MOTOR SKILLS MEANS SPORT IS ACTUALLY VERY HARD FOR HER, AND 2) PROBLEMS WITH COOPERATION AND TEAM WORK. SPORT IS A VERY SOCIAL ACTIVITY AND IT ALSO BECOMES COMPETITIVE IN THIS AGE GROUP AND THE STUDENT MAY BE BULLIED

SUGGESTION: SEE IF THERE IS AN INDIVIDUAL SPORT THE STUDENT CAN DO WELL AT, E.G. RUNNING, OR EVEN GOING TO THE GYM

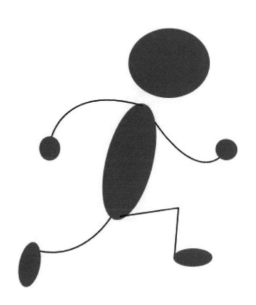

EMOTIONS AND EMOTIONAL MANAGEMENT

FOR CHILDREN WITH ASD, EMOTIONS ARE EXTREME

FOR EXAMPLE, "I'M UPSET WITH YOU" DOESN'T EXIST. INSTEAD, IT'S "LET'S CUT ALL TIES NOW, FOREVER"

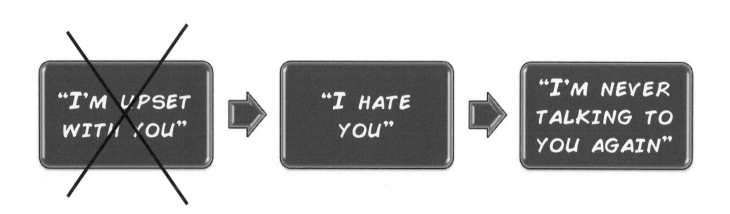

"I'M UPSET WITH YOU" → "I HATE YOU" → "I'M NEVER TALKING TO YOU AGAIN"

THERE ARE SOME STRATEGIES WE CAN WORK WITH TO HELP THEM ASSESS AND IDENTIFY THEIR OWN ANGER LEVELS

The 'Anger Thermometer'

A COLOUR SYSTEM, SUCH AS A THERMOMETER ANALOGY, CAN BE USED TO HELP THE CHILD WITH ASD COMMUNICATE HOW SHE IS FEELING

IT HELPS HER TO IDENTIFY AND SCALE HER OWN ANGER LEVELS

IF SHE IS HAVING PROBLEMS COMMUNICATING HER FEELINGS, HER LOVED ONES CAN SAY, E.G. "ARE YOU FEELING YELLOW?" OR "ARE YOU FEELING ORANGE?" ETC.

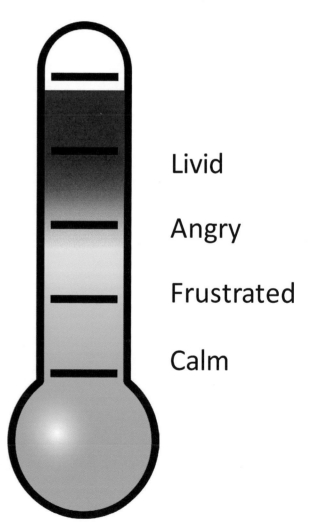

Livid

Angry

Frustrated

Calm

It is important to also help the child link her feelings to situations

So how can we help her to identify the situations that might correspond with each level on the scale?

4. THIS M
ME EXPLO

3. THIS MAKES ME

2. THIS MAKES ME FRUSTRATED

1. THIS DOESN'T BOTHER ME AT ALL

The 'Volcano Concept'

You can relate triggers or situations to this volcano concept. Find out what triggers or situations cause particular negative feelings...

ES

RY

TRIGGERS AT SCHOOL

CREATE A "TRIGGERS AT SCHOOL" TABLE, IDEALLY AT THE BEGINNING OF TERM. THE PURPOSE IS TO MAKE THE TEACHER AWARE OF POTENTIAL TRIGGERS AND THEN DEVELOP SPECIFIC COPING STRATEGIES TO ADDRESS THESE TRIGGERS

	1. THIS DOESN'T BOTHER ME AT ALL	2. THIS MAKES ME FRUSTRATED	3. THIS MAKES ME ANGRY	4. THIS MAKES ME EXPLODE
SOMEBODY SITTING TOO CLOSE TO ME			X	
GETTING MATHS QUESTIONS WRONG		X		
WHEN I DON'T LIKE THE LUNCH AVAILABLE		X		
WHEN FRIENDS WANT TO PLAY SOMETHING DIFFERENT TO ME			X	

TRIGGERS AT HOME

THE SAME THING CAN BE DONE AT HOME, E.G....

	1. THIS DOESN'T BOTHER ME AT ALL	2. THIS MAKES ME FRUSTRATED	3. THIS MAKES ME ANGRY	4. THIS MAKES ME EXPLODE
HAVING TO TURN OFF THE COMPUTER				X
HAVING TO GET DRESSED		X		
BEING TOLD TO HAVE A BATH			X	
WHEN DINNER IS LATE		X		

THIS INFORMATION IS ESPECIALLY IMPORTANT WHEN THE CHILD IS INTRODUCED TO A NEW PERSON, FOR EXAMPLE A SUPPLY TEACHER, A TEMPORARY TEACHER, A NEW TEACHER, A BABY SITTER, A FAMILY MEMBER, ETC...

Lovely things about ASD...

There are lots of assets and lovely things about children with ASD!

What are some lovely things about The Girl with the Curly Hair?

SHE HAS GREAT HOBBIES, E.G., READING

READING

- SHE *HAS TO READ* – TO SAY SHE LIKES IT WOULD BE AN UNDERSTATEMENT

- EVERY NOTICE BOARD, EVERY SIGN, SHE CAN'T WALK PAST WITHOUT READING THEM TOO

- SHE'S HAD "HER HEAD IN A BOOK" EVER SINCE SHE LEARNED TO READ

- SHE MUST TAKE A BOOK *EVERYWHERE* WITH HER

- HER COMPREHENSION OF WRITTEN MATERIAL IS WELL ABOVE AVERAGE

She has lots of love and feels responsible for all animals...

She is very gentle with the cats and talks to them in a very sweet and loving tone of voice. She gives them each a kiss on the top of their head before bedtime

She says she prefers animals to people

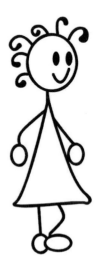

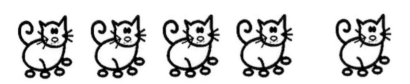

The Girl with the Curly Hair cares a lot about her Mum...

She is always checking that she is OK

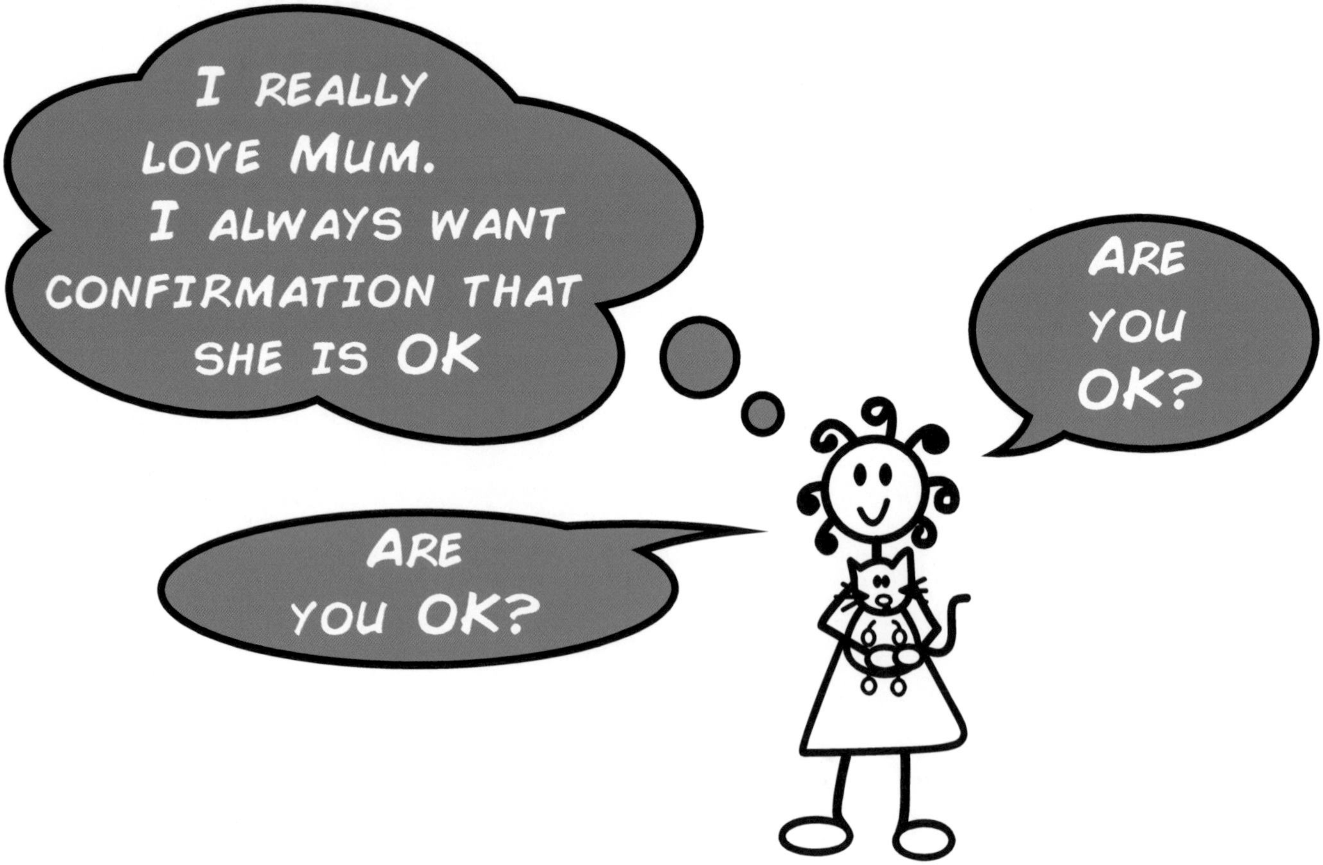

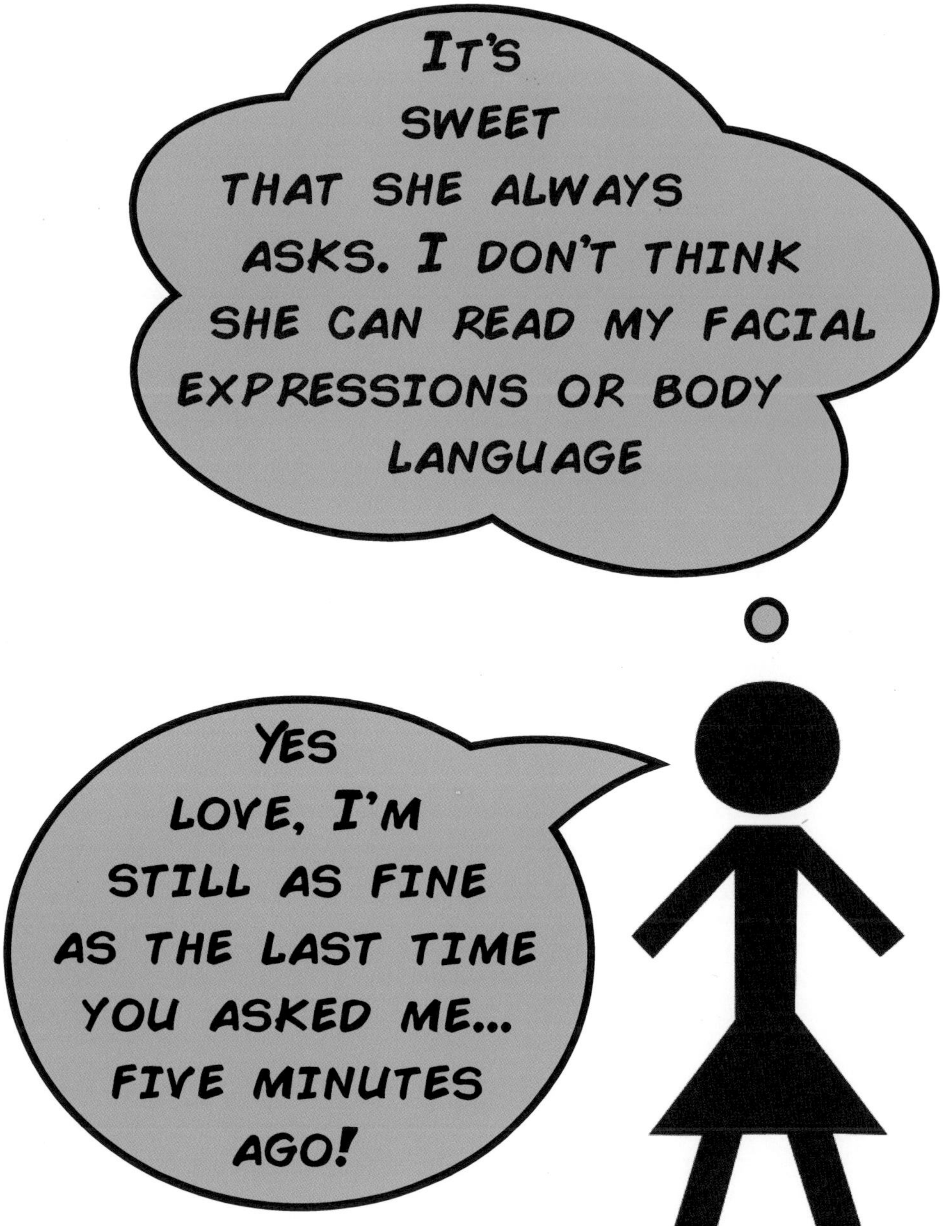
IT'S SWEET THAT SHE ALWAYS ASKS. I DON'T THINK SHE CAN READ MY FACIAL EXPRESSIONS OR BODY LANGUAGE
YES LOVE, I'M STILL AS FINE AS THE LAST TIME YOU ASKED ME... FIVE MINUTES AGO!

To finish...

Be consistent with your rules ("mean what you say and say what you mean", the child with ASD will expect you to keep to your word)

Reward good behaviour, no matter how small

Encourage her at what she is good at

Your child will grow up feeling very happy and very loved with the right adjustments and support

THANKS FOR READING

THIS BOOK WAS INSPIRED BY, AND IS DEDICATED TO, LIAM, (ASD), AGE 8

Other books in The Visual Guides series at the time of writing:

The Visual Guide to Asperger's Syndrome

The Visual Guide to Asperger's Syndrome: Meltdowns and Shutdowns

The Visual Guide to Asperger's Syndrome in 5-8 Year Olds

The Visual Guide to Asperger's Syndrome in 13-16 Year Olds

The Visual Guide to Asperger's Syndrome and Anxiety

The Visual Guide to Asperger's Syndrome for the Neurotypical Partner

New titles are continually being produced so keep an eye out!

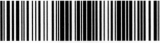

Printed in Great Britain
by Amazon